Naturally Well

Unbeatable Health
The Simple, Sensible Way

Dr. Randall Hardy

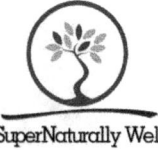

Published by SuperNaturally Well

SuperNaturally Well

6278 N. Federal Hwy. #628
Fort Lauderdale, Florida 33308

www.SuperNaturallyWell.com

Originally published by McClelland and Stewart/Pulse Books 1987

Updated and revised 2011

ISBN: 978-0-9827703-1-3

Library of Congress Control Number: 2010937549

Printed in the USA

This book is dedicated to my late mother and father, Mae and Mac Hardy, who gave me the wisdom to think for myself, and to my beautiful wife Marian, with love. Thanks also to Marian for her editorial content and cover design advice with this revised edition.

Table of Contents

Foreword

There is no question in my mind that we are engaged in a gigantic health experiment with terrible implications. We are eating not only heat-denatured food, but food that is additive loaded and fat, salt and sugar enriched. Some so-called foods are purely chemical substances. We take drugs for anything and everything. We smoke sticks of chemicals and we drink brews that can take rust off a nail. We also breathe in pollution and drink acid rain. And we wonder why we do not feel terrific.

The Baby Boomers are the first-generation heavy users of antibiotics, birth control pills and prescription drugs, and the second generation of people growing up on refined foods. If cancer, arteriosclerosis, arthritis, infertility and diabetes are out of control now, what kind of health future awaits our children and our children's children?

Clearly we must do something. We cannot rely on drugs or surgery to keep us well, or a health care system that treats the dismal end results of long abuse of our bodies.

Dr. Randall Hardy's sound philosophy and common sense suggestions are a solution. We must take them to heart and live them in every detail if we are going to survive.

Carolyn Dean, M.D., N.D.

Carolyn Dean is a medical doctor on the forefront of health issues who has a consulting practice in nutritional and preventative medicine. Dr. Dean has authored or coauthored sixteen books, including *The Everything Alzheimer's Book, Death by Modern Medicine: Seeking Safe Solutions, The Magnesium Miracle, The Yeast Connection and Women's Health, IBS for Dummies, IBS Cookbook for Dummies* and *Hormone Balance.*

Introduction

The Years of Living Dangerously

In the many years since the first edition of *Naturally Well*, things haven't changed that much really. Well, actually they have, but not in the direction I expected events to go—health statistics have worsened. Disease is unchecked despite billions and billions of dollars spent in research and treatment, especially the chronic killing diseases like cancer, heart disease, diabetes and obesity.

We should be healthy. We live longer on the average. Medicine has never been more advanced. Yet, still we worry. A lot. Fear of chronic disease is rampant. Statistics show that cancer strikes one in every three of us. Upwards of fifty percent of us will die of cardiovascular disease. Diabetes is out of control. Obesity is pandemic.

Don't despair. Help is here. There's a simple, healthy and basic way to cope—and it's in this book. It has helped many hundreds of people over the years. So keep reading. It may save your life. One thing's for sure: this book will give you information to change your life for the better.

But don't look for miracles. There aren't any, unless discovering how to be in tune with your own body, learning how to relax and being mindful of what you eat are miracles. In some ways they are.

There are no pills or potions to swallow, no expensive therapies to take. More often than not, the answer to well-being is not just what you do, but also what you don't do—not just what you take, but rather what you avoid. This is the natural way to health. It's the simplest and most affordable too. It can be your way.

I know about the stress you feel. I feel it too. And I've seen it often enough in the countless number of patients and clients I've treated or consulted with in over 30 years as a clinician and health coach. I also know how to reduce stress—by letting the mind-body take care of itself when you give it what it needs. This is only common sense for a fast-track life.

Let me tell you about one of my past clients. John was a typical patient in his thirties with a typical modern lifestyle, and he appeared to be in good health. He told me about his diet and it sounded harmless enough. But his 'minor' and potentially detrimental daily habits examined over a month, astounded him.

The detailed nutritional journal I had him fill out for four weeks revealed the startling truth about his lifestyle. In total, he consumed 60 cups of coffee, 60 teaspoons of sugar, 30 muffins, 60 pieces of white bread, 30 pieces of red meat, 30 to 40 cans of soft drinks, 60 to 90 alcoholic drinks, 240 cigarettes, 60 cookies and 3 pizzas.

John had come to me complaining of morning headaches, irregular bowel movements, indigestion, insomnia, backache and a lack of overall energy.

By simply adjusting John's diet and lifestyle, we were able to eliminate his health issues and put him on the road to vibrant health.

How many of you wake up in the morning feeling as wiped out as you did when you first went to bed? How many of you feel there is something wrong with you, yet you pass a medical exam with flying colors? How many of you are depressed and unhappy?

If you have a chronic illness, are depressed, do not feel well most of the time, or perhaps suffer from frequent flu episodes, colds and other health problems, this book is for you. The suggestions offered in the following chapters have also helped many people overcome serious illness and, most importantly, will prevent many of the diseases so pervasive in our fast-paced world.

One reason I wrote this book is that I want people to begin to have more faith in their bodies' ability to self-heal. People so easily accept medical dogma. And more and more, I'm seeing a population that isn't thinking for itself.

Has blind faith in medical technologies helped create a false sense of confidence that makes us ignore common-sense, responsible limits of the 'good life'? That we will be rescued just in time if we get ourselves into trouble? I think so.

Early indigenous cultures ate food as grown, free of processing and chemicals. Epidemiological studies have shown they had fewer chronic diseases than we suffer from today, despite the lack of advanced medical technology. They understood the intimate connection between the body, the mind and the earth. The earth is our ultimate provider and for countless generations our ancestors knew how to survive and live in harmony with nature.

Throughout history, traditional healing in indigenous cultures has fostered a belief in an inner body intelligence that helped heal both the body and the mind. They viewed this innate wisdom as a mysterious and wondrous companion that animated itself through their physical bodies, their mental capabilities and their emotions.

Although we have tremendous scientific know-how at our disposal, somewhere along the line we have lost that inner knowing, an awareness that recognizes the fundamental laws of nature that govern our physical, emotional and spiritual health. If we are to restore equanimity, we must once again attune ourselves to this ancient genetic wisdom. It's vital for our survival.

We have the choice to synchronize with this inner awareness or fight against it. We have the choice and power to influence our health by being aware of the natural order at work within ourselves and the world around us.

Our responsibility ultimately lies in finding our individual path to wholeness and to pursue it passionately in order to live an optimally healthy life.

Assuming this responsibility is not easy. You'll have to resist the hard sell advertising gimmicks that surround you and reexamine many accepted societal perspectives on health matters. But with time and practice you can stand up for what's best for you. And you will feel better for it.

Our culture accepts chronic disease as normal. You can often hear comments such as: "Everyone I know has some sort of health problem. That's just typical as we age, isn't it?" Society endorses these 'normal' chronic illnesses as part of the human condition and permits mediocre health to be the standard.

This is a profound but not a novel idea, but realize pharmaceuticals can't cure an illness; they only treat the symptoms. Although you may feel better, this is only a temporary fix as long as you continue taking the drug.

Symptoms are an elegant language your body speaks to let you know that something is wrong. They are the body's way of screaming at you for help. Health practitioners can read the signs and symptoms, but only you can hear your bodies 'voice' if you take the time to listen. Once you understand that the message is always 'help and restore me', you must act.

Why should we change our thinking about how we define health? Because our national standards pertaining to health are disgustingly low and that's why so many people are sick. We in the United States have the best medical facilities in the world, which should make ours a healthy continent. Sadly, in fact, the reverse is true. The United Nations and the World Health Organization says the U.S. is dismally low in overall health. Of all the industrialized nations we are said to be far behind.

Obviously we are doing something wrong. Like:

- Eating too much red meat, dairy, sugar and junk food

- Using too many drugs: over-the-counter, pushed or prescribed

- Partying too much

- Sitting around on our backsides

By failing to keep on top of our nutrition, exercise and rest habits, we leave ourselves wide open to disease; in fact, we become a virtual magnet for all sorts of illnesses. For example, there are probably enough bacteria in your mouth at this moment to make you sick if they got out of control, but your body was designed to survive and fight hundreds of daily attacks by these pathogens. We've been taught that bacteria and viruses cause disease, but mostly it's really a malfunction of our immune system that makes us susceptible to all those 'bugs.'

Why should we go through life accepting disease and sickness as normal? It's not natural to have 'ordinary' morning headaches, 'average' menstrual cramps, 'regular' bouts of indigestion, 'typical' acne, and 'usual' arthritic symptoms. Optimal health is our birthright! Our life should be like a candle burning brightly until the end, not sputtering and flickering until it's metaphorically put out by a 'gust of wind.'

The best doctors are the ones who work with the body and allow it to heal itself no matter what the chosen treatment choices. Doctors can't replace or reproduce life. Nobody can. New cells are replacing the dead and sick cells every day. You can help the body continue to create new and healthier cells by eating better, exercising, getting proper rest and developing a positive mental attitude.

Our lives began with the joining of two cells, the sperm and the egg. From this miraculous microscopic organism, the cells divided into two, then four, then sixteen, thirty-two, sixty-four and so on, until a human body with over 50 to 75 trillion cells developed! How did the cells know which ones were to become the kidneys or the liver or the bones or the nervous system?

This inherent wisdom in all living things is so powerful that it created the body and it can heal the body. Do you think it was a mistake the toes on your feet stop growing where they did? We have a pretty smart little body. This inborn intelligence knows more than all the doctors in the world put together! No medical doctor, chiropractor, naturopath or other health practitioner ever cured a disease–it's this powerful life force that heals. The best doctor is the one built right into your own body.

Think about it. If we made an incision in a dead animal, bathed the cut, put cortisone, antibiotics or herbs on the lesion, it would never heal. But if you were to cut your finger, add a medication and bandage it, the medication could help the body heal itself, yet it's the life force in the living body and the wisdom of the immune system that really do the healing. Take the bandage off in a day or two, violà–the wound has healed! Think about how brilliant this body of yours is.

The same idea applies to pathogens in our environment. We might not be able to fight all the bacteria and viruses in the world, but we can increase the resistance of the body to lessen its susceptibility to illness. If we can get the body functioning at its peak level, it will be easier for it to fight disease.

Do you get a headache because of a lack of aspirin in your body? Of course not. Most people have the ability to make every biochemical the body will ever need: antibodies, cortisone, adrenaline, antihistamines and opiates. Many people still blame illness solely on external agents and insist on using only outside interventions to heal themselves. Our dependency on drugs has reached epidemic proportions.

Advertising companies love to play on this ill-founded belief. Some heavyset character on TV says, "I can't believe I ate the whole thing," and immediately pops an antacid. Advertisers are promoting: "Abuse your body. Be a piggy." All you have to do is swallow some pills and you will feel better, they say. Ridiculous, isn't it?

They continue to indoctrinate us into believing that if you have no symptoms, count yourself lucky. If you do have symptoms, pop a pill and you'll be fine. Can't sleep? Take a pill. Feel uncomfortable? Pop another pill. Pills for headaches, pills for menstrual cramps, pills for constipation, pills for indigestion, weight loss and mental depression.

We just simply can't go on this way. What about your kids, your grandchildren? It's a little hypocritical don't you think, to condemn them for 'taking drugs' when they've watched Mom and Dad self-medicate for every little physical and emotional discomfort?

Please remember that I am not criticizing practitioners of emergency medicine. I will most certainly go to the nearest surgeon if I'm ever hit by a Mack truck. I am, however, critical of the practice of medicine in treating the everyday and chronic disorders of the human body with drugs and surgery as routine intervention, while not first considering alternative options such as nutritional guidance and healthy lifestyle management.

But doctors can't take all the blame. Give most patients the choice between a drug or a lifestyle change and you know which option is usually chosen.

Pills won't solve the problem, but education may.

In a report prepared by that *Select Committee on Nutrition and Human Needs* and released by the United States Senate in 1977, entitled *'Dietary Goals for the United States,'* it emphatically stated:

"In all, 6 of the 10 leading causes of death in the United States have been linked to our diet." It went on to say: "Ischemic heart disease, cancer, diabetes and hypertension are the diseases that kill us. They are epidemic in our population. We cannot afford to temporize. We have an obligation to inform the public of the current state of knowledge and to assist the public in making the correct food choices. To do less is to avoid our responsibility."

The report continued:

"There is widespread and unfounded confidence in the ability of medical science to cure or mitigate the effects of such diseases once they occur. Appropriate public education must emphasize the unfortunate but clear limitations of current medical practice in curing common killing diseases. Once hypertension, diabetes, arterial sclerosis or heart disease are manifest, there is in reality very little that medical science can do to return a patient to normal physiological function. As awareness of this limitation increases, the importance of prevention will become all the more obvious."

Right from the horse's mouth. However, if governments constantly give into special interest groups and do not clearly and emphatically convey to the public that a faulty lifestyle can cause illness, they are guilty of neglect. They are contributing to continued widespread suffering and escalating costs in our health care systems for generations to come.

In 2010, the *Report of the Dietary Guidelines Advisory Committee on the Dietary Guidelines for Americans (DGAC), 2010* said we must:

- Reduce the incidence and prevalence of overweight and obesity of the US population by reducing overall calorie intake and increasing physical activity.

- Shift food intake patterns to a more plant-based diet that emphasizes vegetables, cooked dry beans and peas, fruits, whole grains, nuts, and seeds. In addition, increase the intake of seafood and fat-free and low-fat milk and *milk products and consume only moderate amounts of *lean meats, poultry, and eggs.

- Significantly reduce intake of foods containing added sugars and solid fats (SoFAS) because these dietary components contribute excess calories and few, if any, nutrients. In addition, reduce sodium intake and lower intake of refined grains, especially refined grains that are coupled with added sugar, solid fat, and sodium.

- Meet the 2008 Physical Activity Guidelines for Americans.

*Note that I do not recommend dairy products or red meat, but I have included these elements in the report to give you a sense of the authors' overall good intentions.

Continuing, the *DGAC* said:

"On average, Americans of all ages consume too few vegetables, fruits, high-fiber whole grains, low-fat milk and milk products, and seafood and they eat too much added sugars, solid fats, refined grains, and sodium. SoFAS (added solid fats and sugars) contribute approximately 35 percent of calories to the American

18

diet. This is true for children, adolescents, adults, and older adults and for both males and females. Reducing the intake of SoFAS can lead to a badly needed reduction in energy intake and inclusion of more healthful foods into the total diet."

Further in the report, it says:

"The 2010 DGAC recognizes that substantial barriers make it difficult for Americans to accomplish these goals . . . The 2010 DGAC recognizes the significant challenges involved in implementing the goals outlined in this Report. The challenges go beyond cost, economic interests, technological and societal changes, and agricultural limitations, but together, stakeholders and the public can make a difference. We must value preparing and enjoying healthy food and the practices of good nutrition, physical activity, and a healthy lifestyle."

Notice the previous paragraph mentions 'economic interests.' Sadly, there are individuals and corporations who have an investment in keeping us sick. But we can overcome their intent (self-interest) by arming ourselves with knowledge of the right things to do and taking action on them to live a healthier lifestyle based on this knowledge.

We don't need another study to tell us something we and the scientific community have known for years. The basic health recommendations never change—they just make good sense and reinforce the wellness message—but if we don't act on the valuable advice that is given, the consequences will be a harsh reality for those in our society who refuse to heed the warning.

I urge you to change the path you are on if you are off track. Remember, the small incremental changes you make over time, make big differences. For example, walking just 30 minutes every day will give you some noticeable benefits and you will get even better results as you increase the time spent exercising as the days and months progress.

The chapters ahead don't advocate a bizarre, exotic or trendy diet. They don't require you to invest hundreds of dollars in exercise equipment. The approach in this book is based purely on simple common sense that has proven itself over thousands of years.

Don't wait until you are half dead to do something about your health. Read on and you'll turn your body into the ultimate fighting machine!

1

The Proof of the Pudding

Skeptics love to regale me with stories about their 'Uncle Fred.' Fred apparently spends all his time drinking and smoking and carrying on and, amazingly, has never been sick a day in his life. Two years later, you hear that poor Uncle Fred has died of a massive heart attack. Another example: the octogenarians who swear the key to a long life is a few shots of booze each day and a cigar after dinner. We've all heard similar stories.

This just ain't so, folks. At least for most of us. Yes, genetics can protect some people who push the envelope too far, but nature has certain laws. If you break the law, depending on how strong you are—and some people can break the law for a long time—it will eventually catch up with you.

People often brag to me that they haven't been sick in years. I tell them they may have a problem after they confide in me about their lifestyle habits. We look at their diet and it's atrocious: lots of meat, potato chips, doughnuts, chocolate bars and coffee to name a few. To folks who consume foods like these in excess, I say to them there may be trouble ahead if they don't adjust their eating habits. These are the people who may drop dead in two or three years, yet they consider themselves healthy because they haven't had a cold or flu in so long.

Since colds and flu are one way the body rids itself of toxins when immunity has been compromised, the truth is that these people are not even healthy enough to be sick because their bodies don't have the extra energy to dispose of toxic waste. Instead of getting a cold, their bodies spend most of their precious energy resources just trying to neutralize and store away these toxins in body tissues. There is just not enough vitality left in their bodies to cleanse themselves through detoxification (i.e. cold and flu symptoms). You probably haven't heard that before!

As an aside, be aware that as you change your lifestyle for the better, you can sometimes feel worse while you are getting well. In natural healing there is a point reached called the healing crises (or challenge), which is a seeming worsening of your health.

If you start following a proper regime of exercise and diet, you may begin to develop a cold or suffer flu symptoms, your arthritis may worsen or your skin may break out. The specific health problem you want to heal may get worse. Don't let this discourage you! These temporary minor setbacks are just the body's way of self-correcting by ridding itself of toxic waste that has collected in organs and tissues over months and years. It will really depend on how you have lived your life in the past that will determine the nature of the cleansing symptoms and the length of time you experience them.

Here's another—albeit uglier—example. A patient came to see me and he had a horrible ulcer on his leg. He had used cortisone and bandages, but it kept getting worse. I suggested he allow the ulcer to drain because there were a lot of poisons the body was obviously trying to get rid of.

We changed his diet and used an herbal poultice on the ulcer. What came pouring out of this man's leg was all sorts of yellow and green pus, day after day. It was horrid, but at the same time wonderful. As soon as his diet improved and he had cut out sugar and other bad habits, his leg completely cleared up. The body knew, in its own wisdom, that the only way it would allow the ulcer to heal was when the poisons were out of the body. The ulcer was the portal to release the pus and other toxins from the body. Had it been 'plugged', the poisons would've gone deeper perhaps to the kidneys, the heart, or somewhere else in the body.

A woman's menstrual cycle can be considered a positive occurrence too. Every month the body says, "There's a channel of elimination that has opened up again. Let's throw some toxins and waste materials into it." With a change in lifestyle, premenstrual syndrome and so-called normal cramps can disappear because the excess toxic waste that enters the uterus walls through the blood supply has been reduced.

As stated before, we in natural healing consider colds, flu and other minor illnesses a valuable and important way for the body to release toxins. If immunity has been weakened because of stress and toxic buildup, the virus or bacteria multiplies and the body responds appropriately by killing the 'bugs' and eliminating waste products.

That's why it amazes me that people will down massive doses of vitamins the moment they catch a cold. "I stopped the cold," they say, but all they've done is suppress it. Instead of stopping the symptoms, we want to shorten them.

I rarely get colds but if I do, instead of having one for two weeks I have it for a day or two every few years. I don't use vitamins—I adjust my diet. Immediately, I eliminate concentrated foods, eating only fruit, vegetables and soups–the light things. When you have a cold, your body doesn't want to be overwhelmed with many solid foods like meat and junk food. It's saying to you, "I want to use all my energy to throw out toxic waste." If, for example, you were to have a pizza now you might get even sicker. So instead, drink lots of water, steamed and raw veggies and soup, and rest.

Diarrhea is another example of nature cleaning toxins out of the body. By diluting them, it flushes these toxic substances out, quickly and efficiently.

For diarrhea, there are natural remedies to slow it down. Obviously, one wouldn't want to allow dehydration to occur by allowing the diarrhea to go on for too long. But I try to stress to people that diarrhea is a good and natural way for the body to expel toxins. Again, the body in its own wisdom knows what it is doing, so let's not interfere with it.

Fever is another example. When the body is waging a battle with an infection, it has to raise the body temperature to kill the pathogens. So why interfere and decrease it with an aspirin unless absolutely necessary? New mothers are taught to be almost paranoid about minor fever striking their babies, but even a young body knows instinctively how to fight infections and defend itself. Instead, these moms resort to one of several syrups on the market that reduce fevers and suppress the body's chance to fight. Why not lower the fever with a cool bath instead and allow the body to follow its natural instincts? Of course, consult with your doctor if the fevers get out of control.

And cancer. Once considered a chaotic disease, with the tumor growing out of control, researchers are now finding there is some semblance of order in the apparent chaos of cell growth. The body does try to break the tumor down. It tries to kill it. If it can't, it builds a wall around it and keeps it there. That's the body's way of saying, "Let's separate it from the rest of me."

The suppression, controlling or removing of disease symptoms is what we have called healthcare in this country. There are no magic bullets! There are no quick cures. There is no instant health.

Let's say you're driving along in your car and the oil light suddenly comes on. You wouldn't fix it by knocking out the light with a hammer. That's exactly what you do when you take a pill for a headache, for instance. A sick person may fill a prescription at the pharmacy, but two weeks later he's back in the doctor's office feeling worse or complaining of another illness. He's given a different drug. The cycle continues. The doctor never got rid of the illness–he or she just suppressed the symptoms. Eventually this patient may get sicker as a result of not dealing with the cause of his illness.

Symptoms don't always manifest themselves at the level of complaint. Someone, for example, might complain of puffiness under the eyes. In warm weather, her hands and ankles may swell. She starts getting headaches, pain in her lower back and high blood pressure. These are signs and symptoms the body is not well. We soon discover the woman is suffering from kidney problems. So the kidneys are the cause of the symptom complex and once we start healing them, the symptoms will clear up on their own.

Understand your body and what it's saying to you. Disease has a purpose. It's the body's way of fighting to live, and in its fight it manifests symptoms according to the nature of the problem or the toxins in the body or even because of repressed feelings and thoughts in your unconscious.

Recognize that if you spend too much time worrying about getting sick and constantly looking for relief in pills for minor or imaginary illnesses, you can manifest an illness because of the stress you are placing on yourself. It's like trying to avoid a rock in the middle of the road when you're riding your bike. Even though the road is 20 feet wide you manage to hit the rock because you're trying so hard to avoid it. You can attract or create a problem just by paying too much attention to what you fear may happen.

So if, for example, you worry about cancer over and again, maybe the stress can contribute to the cancer. A person who's worried about disease all the time begins to focus on it so much that it can become a reality. They worry, they eat junk to relieve the worry and feel so stressed they don't exercise.

Don't worry. Instead, be smart about what you put into your body and start taking responsibility for your own health without relying heavily on what the advertising and drug industries promote.

Every time you see a doctor and are given drugs is it any wonder your condition doesn't' improve if your lifestyle habits are still the same? If you don't feel well and take pills without dealing with the causes of your problems, you won't be any better off long-term.

Many years ago, I remember a newspaper headline announcing, 'Woman scheduled for heart transplant.' Underneath this was: 'Will be back on beer and pizza soon, doctors say.' That logic is nutty! What caused a heart problem in the first place? Perhaps it was all the beer she drank and the junk food she ate, but sadly, conventional wisdom back then did not recognize the correlation. You'd be surprised even today at the number of people who continue to follow appalling lifestyles while they are trying to recover from life-threatening health problems.

The good news is that people are beginning to refuse prescribed drugs because they're sick of being sick. They are asking their doctors to find other ways to help them, but most traditionally trained medical doctors don't have all the answers. If you look at the course requirements for general practitioners you'll find that doctors do not have enough nutritional instruction during their entire training. Thus the philosophy I'm explaining to you here is alien to some of them.

Fortunately over the years, there have been many doctors receiving education in alternative and complementary health techniques and philosophy in their schools and extracurricular seminars, including nutritional courses. They are the doctors you want to partner with. Doctors like Carolyn Dean who wrote the foreword to this book.

Become an educated consumer. Don't take my word for it. Think it through yourself. Does what I say make common sense? The proof of the pudding is in the eating as the saying goes. It can't hurt you to exercise, relax more and eat better. So try it. If you feel healthier and your symptoms improve, you have proved it to yourself.

The primary reason for the failings within our health system is I'm sad to report, economics. Some people's unquestioning acceptance of our health system has led them to believe that professionals, and the government agencies meant to oversee them, have their best interests in mind. That isn't always true.

History has proven that way of thinking just isn't viable. Follow the money and you will understand why certain policies and procedures are put into place even if they are clearly not in the public's best interests.

In modern times there has been an ongoing hysteria to discover ways to combat disease, and this zeal has resulted in a huge disease industry driven by money and a public fueled by fear.

If you think about it, despite billions of dollars spent every year researching cures for chronic diseases, how many have been discovered so far?

From a holistic perspective of health, using only 'big guns' like powerful drugs, surgery and radiation when lifestyle changes and natural therapies could be helpful or even more effective, just doesn't make sense. It's like burning your house down to get rid of termites. Be aware that there are alternative viewpoints and treatments. Do your research. Become an educated consumer.

You *can* transform your health with a blend of orthodox medicine and natural healing principles, but in this order: lifestyle change and natural remedies, then drugs and surgery if necessary. It really can be that simple for many people depending on the circumstances of the illness.

2

Junk 'n' Jive

Some of the foods people believe to be healthy are, in fact, a contributing cause of many of the chronic degenerative disorders running rampant in our society: cancer, arteriosclerosis, heart disease, osteoporosis, diabetes.

Let's start with *dairy products*–the so-called wonder foods. Over the years, they have received much attention and, no doubt, because they are high in calcium–a bone building agent and purportedly necessary to prevent osteoporosis–a degenerative bone disease.

If we look first to nature for an answer, we discover a high level of calcium in a pasture fed cow that produces milk. Consider its bones, hooves and horns. They show that a proper diet has produced normal, healthy bones. However, the cow doesn't get her calcium from drinking milk; she gets it from eating grass. Isn't it odd to think that we're the only species in the animal kingdom that continues to drink milk after we're weaned?

More and more, I'm finding that the overconsumption of dairy foods is creating a lot of problems, especially in adults who consume milk and cheese frequently. Many of these individuals end up with chronic mucous congestion and other health issues.

Instead of the truth, what we are seeing is the tremendous job that dairy marketing boards across the country are doing of selling their product to a misinformed public.

Having been brainwashed into believing dairy is a wonder food, we've done a great disservice by giving it to children. Clinical evidence has shown over the years that many children who regularly drink milk are chronically sick and suffer from runny noses and recurring ear infections. Take them off milk and you immediately see improvement. You won't have to keep running after them with a tissue.

Instead, give them water with freshly squeezed lemon or lime, herbal teas, vegetable juices and rice milk. If you feel you must give them dairy, it is easier to digest when it's fermented in products like organic yogurt, but in moderation. However, if a child is sensitive to it, skip even this small amount. Remember too, that a baby's best food for the first year of life is human breast milk.

The Physician's Committee for Responsible Medicine in their statement, *Health Concerns About Dairy Products*, said:

"Milk proteins, milk sugar, fat, and saturated fat in dairy products pose health risks for children and encourage the development of obesity, diabetes, and heart disease."

Milk that's whole, organic and unpasteurized, without chemicals and antibiotics, is better for you than regular milk that has only a shadow of its potential nutritional value. Goat's milk is closer to human milk–and is easier on a person's digestive system. However, I recommend that people avoid dairy entirely. Instead have hemp, rice or almond milk–the fresher the better.

Did you know there is an abundance of calcium in other foods? Green leafy vegetables; Swiss chard; spinach, kale, collards and even in tahini butter made from sesame seeds.

And the osteoporosis question hasn't even been dealt with properly.

Did you know that exercise makes bones stronger? You could drink all the milk you wanted, and take your calcium pills, but if you don't exercise, the bones may still become brittle and weak.

If you don't exercise in your 30s and you haven't done much in your 20s, your chances of getting osteoporosis increase dramatically. The solid bone you build now will be solid bone you keep later on. If you haven't done the right things in the past, don't be overly concerned because research has shown that it's never too late to start building and strengthening bone tissue.

On a nation-by-nation basis, people who consume the most calcium have the weakest bones and the highest rates of osteoporosis. The countries with the highest rates of osteoporosis—including the United States—were those in which people consumed the most meat, milk, and other animal foods.

Only in those places where calcium and protein are eaten in relatively high quantities does a deficiency of bone calcium exist. This is due to an excess of animal protein, which can cause a 'leaching' of calcium from the bones. There are other causes that come into play, but I think the conclusion is clear: cut back on animal foods and avoid dairy if you can.

Apart from not being the be-all and end-all of bone building, mass-produced commercial milk is full of chemicals, drugs and hormones and could probably kill the calf for which it was originally intended within months. It wasn't always that way. Fifty or sixty years ago, cows were grazed on wonderfully rich grass and they weren't fed growth hormones and antibiotics.

White flour. It's devitalized 'sawdust' and a waste of money. Nature, in its wisdom, knew exactly what ingredients to put in food. Devitalized white flours with the germ and bran removed have been stripped of more than 70% of their nutrients, including dietary fiber. Food processing destroys much of the goodness. Now, half of the American diet consists of white flour products: bread, cakes, cookies, pastas, pizza, muffins, pies, tortillas. The list is endless.

Advertisers and the companies they represent tell us that certain white breads build strong bodies. But they've enriched the white bread with synthetic vitamins and minerals because they destroyed all the original ones in the whole grain.

Organic food in its whole form is basically perfect. It contains all the vitamins and minerals in a proper balance. When you adulterate, synthesize, hybridize or process food in any way, it automatically becomes foreign and the body may treat it as an invader and create symptoms of rejection such as allergies or rashes.

Simply put, white flour products are difficult for the body to digest. White pizza crust, white bread, doughnuts and such–anything with white flour in it–is hard for the body to break down because it's junk.

If someone consistently loads up on these foods you can imagine the constipation problems they must face. Chew on a slice of white bread and spit it out. What you've got is a big blob of 'gunk' the body somehow has to break down and expel.

In all *grain or cereal products*, go for 100% whole grain. But again, buyer beware. Some of these breads say, for example, whole grain or whole wheat, but look at the label; you can't even decipher the ingredients on the side of the package because there are so many chemicals added.

The best food to buy is that which is easily destroyed by natural exposure. I remember munching on a breakfast cereal one summer when I was a kid. A few bites of that got left on my neighbor's garage floor and they stayed there the whole summer. Even the ants knew better than to eat it.

Vegetables and fruit start to spoil within a few hours of being left on the kitchen counter after being cut. Fresh produce spoils fast. As soon as you find a food that lasts for days and days you know you've got a problem (some packaged foods can last years).

While *eggs* can be an important part of your diet–again, two or three a week–I strongly suggest you buy the organic free-range, omega-3 rich ones. The difference is astounding.

The same holds true for *chickens* (or any fowl). Eat only organic, free-range poultry. It's better for you and the quality of life of the bird! The commercial chickens are being fattened up with chemicals and sold to you as food. Too expensive you say? Eat less of it and enjoy it more. Besides, as the saying goes, what's your health worth to you?

Consistently, I found that many women who suffer from chronic vaginal infections have been virtually given a clean bill of health the moment they remove commercial chicken from their diet. Why? Because the antibiotics ingested by eating chicken kill off the good bacteria in the body and allow the bad ones to grow unchecked and out of control.

Groups of doctors and dentists have become concerned about the antibiotics injected into fowl and other animals because eating these animals builds up a human resistance to the drugs they prescribe. So you can easily grasp that the amount of chemicals given to these birds is astronomical.

Don't feel helpless about the poor food quality you get at your supermarkets. Do something about it. You have choices. Tell them to stock healthier foods or you will go elsewhere to shop. If they refuse, start looking around.

Most health food stores and many grocery chains have free-range chickens and eggs. If you're going for a drive in the country, you might find some there. Ask your local butcher if he's supplying his customers with free-range chickens. These birds are the ones allowed to get their exercise running around the barnyard. They are a healthier bird and they lay healthier eggs. When you eat them, their meat is infinitely better for you.

Red meat (beef including veal, pork and lamb) is another product that's considered by the mainstream health care system to be a vital source of protein. But interestingly, the reported amount of required protein has been declining over the years. That's why getting much of your protein from plant sources is considered to be a wise move by most natural health practitioners.

It takes massive amounts of energy to digest the meat. It hangs around in your gut and begins to putrefy in your intestines. Then it clogs your system with the excess toxins.

Imagine that when you eat a steak and become constipated, it can stay in your system a long time. Take that steak and put it in the oven at 98 °F (your approximate body temperature) for two or three days. Then take it out and see what it looks and smells like. That's the decay that occurs in your body. Not pretty!

People are often told by their doctors that it's perfectly all right to have three bowel movements a week. As long as you're regular, don't worry about it, they say. To me, that's dangerous. I say, rethink that logic. If you stop eating red meat, you'll start to have one, maybe two bowel movements a day, especially with the addition of more veggies, salads, raw nuts and seeds and plenty of purified water and less junk food.

Think about it. If you eat three meals a day, ideally you should have two or three bowel movements a day, depending on the quality of your food. At the very least, you must have one! People who have two or three bowel movements a week are going to have a problem.

Conventional red meat is doctored. It's tainted with agents like carbon monoxide to make it nice and red. In its natural state, meat is a grayish brown color–very unpalatable. Due to stress, there is also a high degree of uric acid released into the animal's tissues at the point of death in the abattoir.

Therefore, I would suggest that you eliminate all red meat from your diet. You'll automatically have more energy and you'll start to feel much better.

So much has been said about the dangers of sugar that I'll just discuss it briefly here.

Sugar–and that includes brown sugar–is devoid of any nutrition. It gives you empty calories. I recommend you use as little as possible and try using agave or stevia as a sweetener instead. This doesn't mean you should add 10 teaspoons of agave into your coffee or tea just because it's better for you. Again, moderation is the key. Try these alternative sweeteners and see if you like them.

Sugar, also called 'white death' by some, is potentially one of the worst foods you can eat. But it's hard to avoid these days because so many foods are loaded with it. The labels on these products may not say 'sugar' but instead you may read something like 'high fructose corn syrup' or 'dextrose', 'fructose' or 'sucrose.' Food manufacturers like to hide this product with jargon so you can't recognize it when you read a label.

The average yearly consumption of sugar was around 4 pounds per person in 1700. These days it's closer to 150 pounds of sugar per person. Can you imagine 150 pounds? Now that's alarming!

Sugar causes an elevation of triglycerides and total cholesterol that can lead to diabetes and cardiovascular problems. Sugar can also cause an overgrowth of fungus and yeast in the body. It depresses immune system function for hours after eating it, thus weakening your resistance to disease. Sugar can initiate a cycle of craving and overindulgence (especially in sweets and processed carbs) and can even result in food binging.

Therefore, reduce your consumption of sugar, especially refined white sugar, its derivatives and all products made with it.

Most canned fruits have been sweetened with sugar. You don't know how long ago the fruit was picked and preserved and its nutritional value is zilch.

Numerous large food chains are changing their approach to food marketing. Some foods are now sold without chemicals or preservatives. Various stores display a regular store item alongside its natural counterpart, so you can buy ketchup with sugar or ketchup without, children's treats with sugar, children's treats without. The consumer is getting more of a choice.

Most big corporate grocery stores are not doing this out of principle or concern for your health. They're doing it because the consumer is demanding it and the store is cashing in on the demand.

That's why I always first recommend you buy from small business owners in the natural health field. Most exhibit consciousness and heart while serving their customers. (Just for the record, I have also met wonderful employees of larger corporations who really do care about the welfare of their customers too).

Fresh vegetables and fruit represent food in its whole form. Try to buy the freshest fruits and vegetables possible, preferably those grown organically. If you can't get to a farmer's market or supermarket that has a good turnover of fresh fruits and vegetables, then frozen ones are the next best thing.

If you can, research local growers, farmer's markets and suppliers of organic food. Many will deliver a box of seasonal organic produce to your door right from the field.

Take advantage of the power you ultimately have as a consumer and buy the best foods that you can. Support those people and companies committed to growing the purest, healthiest foods.

3

Bull for Breakfast

A former patient of mine was a graduate student at the Royal Conservatory of Music. He had bad nodules on his fingers, much like rheumatoid arthritis. As a pianist, his hands were the key to his career, but his doctors feared for his future and suggested that drugs and surgery were the only options to correct his disorder.

Thanks to natural healing principles, he's still playing the piano and his hands are in perfect condition.

How did I help him? Primarily by changing his diet. It turned out that red meat had contributed to an inflammation of the synovial capsule around the joints, so naturally we eliminated the meat. But then we also discovered that our pianist had a fondness for coffee, sugar and chocolate. By getting rid of all of these offending foods in his diet, we were able to restore the intelligent life force in this man's body and clear up some potentially dangerous symptoms. When he switched to herbal teas the healing was further sped up.

Nutritious food can prevent illness, and it makes sense that if you keep junk food out of your body you'll be a healthier person for it. Not only will this prevent illness, it will, from what I have seen for over 30 years, start to reverse many of the chronic illnesses such as cardiovascular disease, diabetes and obesity.

The standard food fare for many people–cheeseburgers, fries and milk shakes–satisfies the nutritional quota for the basic food groups set out in some older food guides. However, the meat is filled with hormones and chemicals, the white buns contain sugar, the French fries are drenched in salt and saturated fat and the milkshakes, well, remember what I said about dairy in the previous chapter?

This is a dangerous diet. It's no wonder kids are having hamburger attacks–they're addicted! This food is designed to create a desire for more of it. And to add insult to injury, many leading US hospitals are contracting fast food companies to provide their catering services, a move which sends a mixed message about healthy eating. Many children's hospitals have affiliation with and corporate sponsorship from junk food companies and serve this stuff to sick kids. As I said earlier, the medical establishment has a lot to learn when it comes to nutrition.

Many people's bodies are numb from eating too much junk food; they wouldn't know if the foods they eat are causing adverse reactions because the body purposely diminishes sensation when constantly eating things like red meat, sugar, dairy, white flour products and drinking too much alcohol. It doesn't want to feel the hurt. Drugs taken for symptoms that do manage to get through can further distort the true picture of their health. Many people believe that they are healthy when their bodies have just given up telling them that they are not. A short-term cleansing program will help correct the problem.

A cleansing diet helps people reach a finely tuned state. For example, if after a cleansing program someone eats a steak and a chocolate bar, suddenly they feel terrible, even if they regularly indulged in these foods before the cleanse. This gives people firsthand knowledge about the impact these kinds of foods are having on them. They learn what to avoid and what their bodies will tolerate and more importantly, thrive on, because it is now more sensitive and responsive to everything eaten.

If you admit to being a junk food junkie–most of us have succumbed to that addiction at one time or another–and are ready to detoxify the body, here are a few easy to follow pointers.

Eating vegetables, veggie based soups and salads, small portions of grain like quinoa (with a drizzle of extra virgin olive oil) and green veggie juices is a simple but effective cleansing diet. It helps people change their eating habits and detoxify their bodies. The first and most exciting thing this program does is help people lose weight quickly without sending them into a frenzy of starvation. They get enough food and proper nutrition and they feel good knowing their body is healing itself.

I dislike giving meal plans because no one likes to follow them. They are too rigid. But if you need some guidelines here is what I recommend:

The 10 Day Naturally Well Cleansing Program:

1. Steamed or raw vegetables with quinoa, brown rice or lentils, seasoned with cayenne pepper, a no salt herbal seasoning, garlic and ginger. You can add a drizzle of extra virgin olive oil as well. The portion ratio is 75% veggies and 25% grain or lentils. You may add a side salad as well with olive oil, lemon juice and seasoning. Have this for lunch and dinner.

2. You can have the above for breakfast if you like, but you'll probably prefer a bowl of fresh low sugar fruit such as berries, peaches, plums and apples with almond, hemp or rice milk. To this you can also add a tablespoon of organic ground flax seeds.

3. A baked sweet potato is also allowed at dinner. You can also add a small bowl of veggie soup if you feel hungry at lunch and dinner.

4. Drinking a freshly made vegetable 'green' drink made in a juicer or bought at the local juice bar and added to your cleansing program (at least every other day), is good for you. It floods the body with alkaline phytonutrients. You can use most vegetables for your drink with a little added beet and carrot and flavored with ginger and garlic.

Once again, the bonus is that you'll lose weight if you need to and you won't have to worry about counting calories or grams of fat.

After 10 days, or should you decide to bypass the cleansing program altogether, you can start using the *'Naturally Well Nutrition and Lifestyle Guidelines'* beginning on page 44, a common sense long-term lifestyle program anyone can follow.

If you suspect you have specific food allergies or intolerances, I often suggest that a person test for them by reintroducing a single new food a day into the diet after the cleansing program.

If any food is a problem for you, symptoms can occur immediately, in the middle of the night or the next morning. Look for any new symptoms that present themselves such as a cough, sneezing, itchy or puffy eyes, indigestion and bloating or even headaches. See if some of your old symptoms reoccur. If any particular food bothers you, avoid it. The cleansing diet tunes people in to their bodies and they begin to observe how it responds. Keeping a food journal to record physical and emotional symptoms is very helpful in identifying food intolerances.

For longer term health maintenance, I suggest that you follow a lifestyle program that is highly alkaline-forming in the body (as opposed to acid-forming) and low in sugars. I will go over this outline in more detail in another book, but allow me now to give you more clarity on this particular point.

Foods that make the body tissues most acidic are meats (especially red meat), white sugar and white flour and all products made with them, sodas, dairy, coffee, alcohol, fried and junk foods. Excessive worry and tobacco products can also create increased tissue acidity.

When the body becomes too acidic, nutrient transport and oxygen exchange in the cell becomes impaired. You feel tired and listless. Most importantly, chronic low-grade metabolic acidosis can lead to a state of local or widespread inflammation in the body that doesn't go away. Research has shown that longstanding inflammation can lead to many of the chronic (and killing) diseases we suffer from today, including obesity.

In order to buffer the acids in the body we must eat enough alkalizing foods—veggies, salads and low sugar fruit—and drink pure water. Ideally, we must eat *mostly* high water content alkalizing foods to stay healthy.

For example, at meals have at least 50% (preferably 75%) of your plate filled with veggies. Then, a small portion (25%) of your plate can be one of the following: fish or fowl, a whole grain or beans or eggs. Try to incorporate at least 15 vegetarian-only meals a week into your diet.

Eat low sugar fruits such as berries, apples, pears, plums and cherries—your northern grown fruits. Tropical fruits such as pineapple, mango, papaya and bananas are high in sugar. Eat these foods infrequently.

This way of eating, with a minimum 6–8 glasses of purified water daily, will help keep your body in the correct pH range (slightly alkaline), reduce or eliminate inflammation and lessen the frequency of illness, both acute and chronic.

The Naturally Well Nutrition and Lifestyle Guidelines

1. Eat only natural foods whenever possible. They should be whole, unprocessed and unrefined. Try to eat foods in season, as grown.

2. If possible, eat organic foods whenever you can. Avoid foods with chemicals, preservatives and additives. A good general rule of thumb is this: if you can't pronounce the ingredients listed on the package of a product, don't buy it. It's best to avoid as much packaged food as possible.

3. Avoid an excess of animal protein in your diet. Avoid red meat entirely (any meat except fish or fowl). If you eat fish or fowl, limit them to two or three times a week in total. Buy organic free-range fowl and wild-caught fish. Eat only 2 or 3 organic eggs a week.

4. Eat only when you're hungry. Nature has provided you with a built-in mechanism within your brain that will tell you precisely when you should eat or drink (when in doubt drink a glass of

water. Often we mistake hunger for thirst). Follow your own hunger and thirst signals (unless you are craving an addictive substance). Food eaten without an appetite will overburden the digestive organs.

5. Eat slowly in a relaxed, unhurried atmosphere. Slow mindful eating and thorough chewing are essential to good digestion. Enjoy the food you eat.

6. Eat several small meals a day rather than three large meals if you can.

7. Do not mix too many foods at the same meal. The fewer foods you mix, the better your digestion will be.

8. Don't mix fruit with any other food. Fruit spends less time in the stomach than other foods and if eaten with or immediately after a heavy meal, fermentation and gas (bloating) can occur. Eat fruit twenty minutes before anything else and at least one hour after a meal, especially if you have digestive problems.

9. Practice systematic under eating. Push yourself away from the table before you feel full. Avoid eating after 7 p.m.

10. Drink water that is as pure and natural as you can find. Do not drink with meals because doing so can potentially dilute the digestive acids in the stomach. You will also avoid the tendency to 'wash down' your meals instead of chewing your food. Consume liquids half an hour before or after meals.

11. Drink a freshly made glass of 'green juice' prepared with kale, organic beet tops, celery, cucumber, carrots, beets, parsley, a little ginger and garlic, etc. Having this drink made in a juicer or blender that keeps some or all the fiber is beneficial.

12. Ditch the following health destroyers:

- Tobacco, including cigars

- Red meat

- Refined white sugar, white flour products and everything made with them: bread, pastry, packaged cereals, pies, doughnuts, ice cream, candy, cookies, gum, etc.

- Artificial sugars and fake fats (interesterified fats)

- Dairy products

- All processed, refined, canned or factory made foods

- All fried foods

- Milk chocolate (dark chocolate is acceptable occasionally)

- Mustard, black and white pepper (use cayenne pepper), white vinegar

- Too much iodized table salt (use unprocessed sea salt instead and sea vegetables for iodine)

- Coffee, non-herbal tea (except a little green tea), soft drinks

- Alcohol (two or three drinks a week may not hurt if you are healthy, but be careful not to develop a dependency)

- All chemical drugs (pushed or prescribed), except in an emergency and only when prescribed by a doctor

- An ongoing negative attitude

- A lazy life

Keep a weekly lifestyle and food journal for a few months to help you observe your exercise and nutritional patterns. It can be very revealing.

By following these simple guidelines you'll gain a well-balanced lifestyle and avoid what I term 'nutritional neurosis.' This occurs when one is so preoccupied following endless fad diets that they miss out on having fun.

Experiment and enjoy!

4

Wired for Life

At one time or another, most of us have entered the 'twilight zone', that state of oblivion you reach when you've had one too many drinks, tokes or snorts. Some of us go on a food binge and fall into the 'food coma.'

Experiencing the twilight zone and the food coma are your body's way of telling you that you've just stepped over the moderation line and into the danger zone.

The moderation line is the point up to which your body will accept being assaulted before it sounds the alarm. It's like having your best friend rescue you before you make a complete idiot of yourself. And if you fail to call it quits at that time, you're on your own and are in serious danger of damaging yourself—perhaps irreparably over time.

The real cause of this destructive behavior is that in truth your brain is just trying to change your emotional state—one that may be angry, upset, afraid, frustrated or even feeling unloved—to one that feels better, even temporarily. The brain's goal is to get a break from the stress. If you received comfort, consolation and pleasure from a handful of chocolates or a few glasses of wine during prior emotional upsets, the brain linked this 'feel good' sensation to the eating and drinking and therefore repeats it over and over again to get the same relief: a temporary diversion from reality.

Jeannie thinks her five coffees a day are just a way to get her going in the morning and keep her 'up' throughout the day. Bob believes his daily martinis at lunch relax him and give him enough confidence to make that big sale. Susie only gets a good night's sleep with the aid of a sleeping pill. All these people need their little 'fix' to get them through the day, and thus they are all hooked to some extent.

Although the cigarette calmed your nerves, the morning coffee helped you wake up, or the martini at lunch helped your shakes, the truth is that your body has begun to depend on these substances to establish and uphold physiological and psychological equilibrium.

It doesn't surprise anyone today when it is mentioned that many substances such as caffeine, nicotine and alcohol can cause damage to the body over years of abuse and that they all lower the body's ability to fight disease.

Alcohol

As with other drugs, the dangers of alcohol have been reiterated in anti-alcohol advertising campaigns and media reports. Alcohol is creating distressing statistics among young and old alike. Again, if you can handle it without abusing it, okay, but it's as deadly as a snake bite if you can't.

Research shows that people who become addicted to this socially acceptable drug are not moral degenerates, but in fact may be heirs to a genetic propensity for addiction. In other words, some people are born not to drink. Ever. If you feel you are beginning to tolerate larger amounts of alcohol, drink alone and see personality changes, get help.

Don't be fooled by the classic Hollywood image of an alcoholic; you don't have to do a face dip to the pavement every night to have a problem. Even those who have two or three drinks a day but need and crave it are alcoholics.

While the helping professions stress the dangers of excessive alcohol consumption, society continues to put an even heavier pressure on us to drink. It's part of being social, we're told.

You can be sociable and safe at the same time; non-alcoholic beer and wine are now sold in grocery stores almost everywhere. Some people just camouflage their drinks. I know one person who throws a couple of ice cubes into a glass of apple juice at a party and it looks just like scotch or rye.

Don't feel self-conscious about this. The only person who's going to look after your health is you. You'd be surprised at the number of people who are eliminating alcohol without anyone being the wiser.

I needed to stop drinking years ago; I did it and so can you.

Cigarettes

This year, cigarettes will contribute to the deaths of over one million people in North America. It is a well-established fact that smokers significantly increase their chances of getting sick. Just read any medical text or search the internet. Tobacco use accounts for at least 30% of all cancer deaths and 87% of lung cancer deaths, not to mention the devastating effects of second hand smoke on innocent bystanders.

Along with poor lifestyle habits, tobacco contributes to elevated cholesterol and plaque deposits in your body's arteries.

Quitting will take effort, determination and all the 'grit' you can muster, but it will be worth it. Also, by following the lifestyle changes recommended in this book, you will not gain significant weight when done in tandem!

Caffeine

Coffee has been cited as a cause of cystic breast disease in women. Caffeine has also joined the list of substances thought or known to increase the risk of cancer.

The caffeine that is found in coffee, tea, colas, cocoa preparations, chocolate and many pain remedies causes blood sugar levels to drop, resulting in fatigue and irritability. Over-consuming caffeine can also create symptoms of anxiety, poor concentration and sleeplessness.

Just because coffee is widespread and part of your daily rituals doesn't mean it's good for you. Do you get headaches or feel terrible upon stopping coffee for a day or two? Aren't these symptoms a warning that caffeine is much more habit-forming than you may be comfortable admitting? When you withdraw a food, beverage or substance from the body and you experience adverse symptoms, isn't this like an addiction? I guarantee if you stay away from carrots for a few days you won't get a headache! That's a clue.

Contrary to popular belief, I have found that coffee is one of the easiest of all addictive substances to let go of once you get over a few days of feeling poorly as the body eliminates this toxin. Withdraw gradually to avoid a potential monster headache.

Marijuana

Judging from the marijuana users that I have treated in my practice, I found that those who used marijuana several times a day for years had a real problem with memory loss and dealing with reality. Some of them had problems getting things done or just following through with day-to-day activities. The mood swings could be problematic as well.

Many people smoke pot these days. I understand the lure: zoning out and getting away from stress can be tempting. However, if you already find it tough coping with everyday life–and who doesn't these days–imagine the mess you'll find yourself in if you start depending on this drug.

Some people have an addictive personality to begin with. Give them something new to try and they're hooked for life.

Unlike alcohol, there is no way you can become physically dependent on pot. However, the psychological reliance it creates has been clinically documented. This is a drug that can be abused because of its relaxation effects.

In terms of physical hazards, marijuana gives you the same smoke residue that you get with cigarettes. Habitual pot smokers can develop that wheezing sound most people associate with heavy tobacco use–a buildup of mucus causing lung congestion and sinus problems.

If you were to put a tissue over a cigarette and smoke it you'd be horrified at the amount of residue that collects in the tissue. You get that same toxic residue from pot.

If there's a positive side to marijuana it's that it doesn't hit you the same way alcohol does. A person could have a few tokes, get a little high and be silly; a person who has four or five beers can tend to get pretty obnoxious the more he drinks. The personality changes are more dramatic in people who drink than they are in people who smoke pot. Alcohol can induce mental instability and depression in some people.

Cocaine

Many of the chronic abusers I used to treat as a clinician were habitual cocaine users.

There was a time when I would ask all the kids I'd treat for various disorders if they did coke. Later, I was asking the same question of the Wall Street brigade.

The physiological toll cocaine takes has also extended itself to heart problems—namely cocaine induced heart failure, which should be reason enough to stay away from it.

The abuse of other drugs is rampant too: methamphetamine, ecstasy and opiates for example. Education about the potential harm of these substances is important, but not enough. We also need to educate ourselves about the dangers of misusing overprescribed sedatives and antidepressants.

The cumulative effect of these addictive substances will surprise you when you calculate your daily consumption of caffeine, nicotine, alcohol, marijuana and prescribed drugs, for example. Multiply by 365 for a year's total. The stress created on your body's immune system, not to mention your liver and kidneys, is tremendous.

The good news is that I have seen many people break their unhealthy habits by following the suggestions in this book. Your body, with its amazing healing powers, will begin to excrete the accumulated toxins. As your system purifies itself, you will lose much of the physical craving that once enslaved you. You will be free!

There are also many centers that are established to help you deal with hard addictions. Get help at professional centers where you feel most comfortable with their approach and philosophy.

5

Use It or Lose It

The importance of exercise can't be emphasized enough and still people refuse to set aside a few hours a week and give their bodies a break in routine.

There are valid reasons for exercising—mainly, your life depends on it. Perhaps this chapter will convince you.

Inside the body, there is a network of conduits that circulate just like a winding river moving one way toward the heart. This 'river', known as the lymphatic system, acts like a collecting sewage system that carries away waste materials.

The lymphatic system is an intricate, delicate network that moves throughout the body from head to toe. Glands (collecting areas, out-pockets of the lymph system) are located in the neck, chest, abdomen, groin and armpits.

If there's too much waste material in the lymph system, the body has nowhere to put it. It's like having too many logs in a river; some will eventually sink to the bottom and just stagnate, clogging the river.

The body relies on muscle contraction to squeeze the waste material through the lymphatic system. If a person doesn't exercise, you begin to understand why he becomes lethargic and 'lumpy.' He's piled up too much garbage in his body and it's just sitting there. When you exercise, the muscles pump the lymph fluid, moving the contained waste material along to various channels of elimination.

Just as exercise starts up this lymph mechanism, it also increases blood circulation. People who complain of cold hands and feet–even in warm weather–have a problem with their circulation. This could also show problems with the thyroid and adrenal glands and exercise will help these conditions too.

There was a time when cardiologists prescribed lengthy bed rest for cardiac patients. Now they're putting the same patients into a cardiac rehab exercise program. The heart, like any other muscle in your body, needs regular exercise to keep it strong and healthy.

Sometimes it takes a heart attack to shake someone up to the fact that that they're just not living right. But doesn't it make sense to reduce the odds before it's too late? Don't wait for a heart attack to change your lifestyle. If you've had a heart attack, count yourself lucky that you survived it. Recognize where things went wrong. Okay. So you blew it. You overindulged in questionable food, you may have smoked and you didn't exercise enough. When you exercise, you place demands upon your body including the heart. It will respond to this demand by getting stronger.

An added benefit of exercise is that it increases your mental well-being because oxygen-filled blood is moving to the brain.

Your body is a very sensitive machine and if it's listless due to lack of exercise (and eating junk food), you can't possibly know what you are feeling: physically tired and or just bored, or both. In addition to a good diet, exercise heightens awareness of your body's true state.

For example, people often say to me that they're too tired to exercise, and I ask them what that tiredness is like: are they bored or weary? If they answer they are exhausted, I ask them how they would feel about going to an exciting movie, theater performance or sports event that evening, doing something that would really interest them. If they perk up and start to feel better, the tiredness is obviously partly due to being in a mental rut.

Start your exercise program out slowly and see just how you feel. Then get out and have some fun. Both exercise and outings will give you more zest for life!

The best thing about exercise is that it gives you an immediate return on the time invested in it. You feel better instantly.

Psychologically, exercise is wonderful. If you're ever angry or upset, go for a run or a brisk walk; you'll feel much better after you've rid yourself of the emotional tension.

Exercise is such an inexpensive way to stay healthy and prevent disease. I'm not asking you to take out an expensive membership in a health club or to buy fancy equipment (but you could!). All you need is a pair of shorts, a pair of running shoes and a skipping rope.

Start by skipping rope a few minutes a day. Your feet and hands won't be as cold. Your digestive system will improve. If you suffer from constipation, you'll find that exercise will often clear it up. Exercise also reduces tension and stress.

People who don't watch what they eat but play squash four or five times a week are not going to suffer in the same way couch potatoes do, because their body is constantly moving dietary indiscretions through elimination channels more efficiently.

You may be surprised to hear me say this, but I would rather see someone eat an inferior diet and exercise like crazy than to eat properly and not exercise at all. It's that important. Please understand this is not what I am suggesting–one needs proper balance–hopefully you understand the point I am making.

It amazes me how lazy people have become; they sit in a chair and order their spouse to get them a beer or a sandwich. To them I say, get it yourself! To people who literally drive the two minutes to the corner store I say, leave your keys at home and walk! To the busy executives who complain about not having enough time to exercise I say, buy a skipping rope, put it in your briefcase and skip in the privacy of your office every day or walk at lunchtime. Use stairs instead of the elevator. Do whatever it takes.

So often we get caught up in our work, with all the tension and stress it causes, without taking the time to release this burden. Try to exercise three times a week and do something that increases your circulation and induces perspiration; do 10 push-ups, skip rope, take yoga or tai chi classes, swim, play tennis, ride a bike, walk around the block or stretch. There are so many enjoyable things to do.

Office workers–from corporate executives to secretaries–sit at their desks for hours in a groggy state, finding it hard to concentrate or to get motivated to complete assignments. With regular exercise, your work will improve. You will notice greater mental clarity and having more energy. And you'll also have more energy to enjoy your family and friends in leisure time as well.

How about buying a mini-trampoline that you can store under your bed or in your closet? Are you able to get up 15 minutes earlier in the morning and bounce on it while listening to your favorite music or audio program? I bet you can! It also has the added benefit of being one of the best exercises for the lymph system.

Don't confuse work with exercise. Confidential to homemakers and weekend handymen: cleaning your house or fixing the toilet is not exercise–its work. Many people believe they get plenty of exercise running up and down the stairs after the kids, washing dishes, vacuuming, cutting the lawn. Housework doesn't increase the heart rate the same way as a game of squash does. Housework is low-level activity that doesn't sufficiently exercise the body, the heart muscle and the lungs. But it's still better than nothing.

The discipline of maintaining regular exercise is wonderful for self-esteem because you're following through on a commitment you made to yourself, even though you may not feel like doing it every time. As a result, your resolve is strengthened. This sense of personal empowerment carries over into other areas of your life too.

There's no excuse not to exercise. Sign up for one of the low cost programs offered by churches, recreation or community centers. Start working out with your favorite video or TV exercise guru each day.

Play with your kids. Race with them, set up 100 yard dashes. Enjoy a game of soccer or football with them. Get your children involved in a fitness activity. Be a role model!

Exercise has to be intentional and enjoyable and you have to be committed to it. If you're not really into it, you won't stick with it.

Exercise and nutrition go hand in hand: people cut out their bad habits more easily and their eating improves as they become increasingly active.

We've all seen people who want to lose weight or quit a habit. They go through the motions without making a real commitment and therefore they don't succeed. However, once someone truly commits to being healthy through exercise, they will incorporate it into their schedule and find at least 30 minutes a day to work at it. The time spent exercising will increase once it's a firm habit and you begin to feel better. But first, make a lasting promise to yourself to be healthy.

People who exercise regularly feel energized. They go to bed feeling good and they easily fall into a wonderfully deep sleep.

6

ZZZZZZ–Deep Sleep–Cheap

A good night's sleep is as rare these days as insider tips on Wall Street.

If you're having trouble getting to sleep at night, or if you put in eight hours of sleep but wake up feeling as if you've had only eight minutes, you're not alone.

In a society that expects top performance and top speed, it's no wonder that insomnia and many other sleep disorders are so prevalent.

Our bodies cannot achieve proper rest when we are constantly 'wired up.' We are overstimulated due to stress and a high intake of sugar, junk food, cigarettes, additives and coffee; all of these consumed chemicals create a state in which the body's 'alarm system' is continually on.

Let's look at the body's alarm mechanism for a moment.

If you were chased by a huge grizzly bear you'd either fight or you'd run. That's the way the body's alarm is set up. It's either wired up for a battle or it's disconnected.

The body doesn't know the difference between the real emergency (the bear, in this case) or something you stress about (your report that's due on Monday morning).

Here's another example. If you and I are watching a movie and one of the characters is about to be engulfed by a giant squid, our logical brain tells us it's only a movie, but our body doesn't know the difference. It reacts as if we are witnessing a terrible incident. If we hooked you up to monitoring equipment we could measure the reaction: pupils dilate, the skin pores open, you begin to sweat and your respiration rate increases. These are all the physiological responses that happen in a true emergency.

In the real world, we encounter many mini-stresses each day and they become so commonplace that we accept them as normal:

You get up in the morning to the sound of the kids screaming for their breakfast and you go into this stress mode.

You get to the bus stop and the bus goes right by you, splashing water all over you.

You get to work and the boss starts yelling at you because you're ten minutes late.

And on it goes.

Your body gets conditioned to go into this state of anxiety and over time, the alarm stays on.

That is what's meant by being constantly 'wired.' And that's why you may complain of being tired all the time because you're always stressed out. Try to be mindful of the relationship between chronic exhaustion and stress.

What happens is that throughout the day as you face the stresses, your muscles are constantly ready to 'fight' and eventually the muscles begin to fatigue.

Lactic acid is a byproduct of muscle tension. When you do physical activity, the lactic acid is squeezed into the bloodstream and disposed of properly. But if you're just sitting there thinking stressful thoughts and worrying, the muscles fire and the lactic acid just pools there. This increase of acid in the body is one reason you feel tired.

That's why exercise is important, because it provides a release for the buildup of tension and clears away lactic acid accumulation.

In addition, if you don't exercise, you can end up with sore, tense muscles. If someone were to touch you on the shoulder you go through the roof because the muscles had become inflamed with lactic acid—it's called myofascitis. This can also be one of the factors that lead to fibromyalgia.

I'll bet the majority of you reading this are recognizing yourselves in this chapter!

To reiterate some of the previous ideas already discussed:

You come home from work after an exhausting day's worth of mini-stresses. Your mind can't shut off. Your body can't shut off. It doesn't know how to return to a normal state.

But in our high-tech everyday world, the alarm is always on, and you never know what it's like to be relaxed. In our fast-paced life, many of us live in a mini-state of fear, anxiety and insecurity.

When living with this constant stress, breathing patterns can become very shallow, like the breathing you do when you're afraid.

Clearly, if you display the signs and symptoms I have discussed so far, it's time to learn how to manage and respond to stress in healthy ways.

Many of us have the tendency to burn the candle at both ends. I did it, and I know that when I was younger I could work around the clock and then party all night. But at some point in our lives the body says, "That's it. No more. Time to slow down." That point is usually reached when we turn 30, though most of us don't listen. Most people under the age of 30 can go on overtime because of their youthful vigor and vitality and not need much rest. After age 30, it all changes. More rest is vital, including the quality and quantity of sleep. Some people may need six hours' sleep. Others may need 9 hours. Whatever your requirements, get a good start to your day by getting out of bed as soon as you wake up.

Another good tip is the more sleep you get before midnight, the better it is for you. If you went to bed at 2 a.m. and woke up at 10 in the morning, you probably wouldn't feel as refreshed as someone who went to bed at 10 p.m. and woke up at 6 a.m.

People who work night shift for years can potentially experience several health problems because their bodies are out of sync with nature's cycles. We are biologically programmed to go to bed when the sun sets and to rise at daybreak.

So, a person who sleeps all day and works all night is just throwing his whole biorhythm out the window because the body is attuned to these body cycles. We are programmed to sleep and eat at specific times.

Of course, shift work has become a reality in the workplace and if you are one of those people who must work nights, you have to be especially cautious when it comes to your lifestyle.

Police officers and nurses, anyone who works nights, can get used to this reversed schedule, but they are setting themselves up for future grief if they don't maintain proper rest, nutrition and exercise habits.

Sometimes shift work is unavoidable, but if you make a commitment to be healthy, there are ways of reducing the risks of body breakdown. For example, rather than relying on doughnuts and coffee, pack a healthy lunch and snacks to get you through the night. Schedule regular exercise periods during the week to keep your body from getting sluggish. Getting regular massage and bodywork is helpful as well. And as this chapter urges, get the proper rest. It's vital for maintaining such a rigorous schedule.

Because there's been so much emphasis lately on the importance of relaxation, we often try too hard. It's like someone trying desperately to sleep. They lie in bed, eyes wide open (or forced shut) trying to convince themselves they will relax and they will sleep. And yet they never get to sleep.

The body knows how to sleep if you just leave it alone. As I have said in previous chapters, the body knows, in its own wisdom, how to get rid of infections and viruses. It knows how to heal itself. So, too, the body knows how to put itself into a state where it can relax and sleep. Look at children: they play, they lay their head down and they fall sleep just about anywhere.

Just as a healthy body knows when to get up, it also knows, intuitively, when it wants to sleep. If you're not tired at night because you feel stressed, then do something; walk around, do the dishes, clean the floor, read a book, anything to drain off the mental overload that may be causing you to feel wired up.

Some people need a ritual preparation to relax; for example, a long, warm aromatherapy bath by candle light. Do anything healthy that will slow the body and the mind down.

Another technique is self-induced relaxation. The 'Naturally Well Relaxation Technique' on the next page is simple to do.

This exercise puts your mind into a light state of alpha (the same state you're in when you're watching a mindless, boring TV program). If you can relax yourself to the point where brain wave activity begins to slow down enough, you can achieve maximum deep sleep. It will take some practice, but learning how to relax the mind and body is well worth the time invested.

This procedure works best if you can keep yourself calm throughout the day and not 'wig out' or get super-stressed. When you go to bed, with suggestions from this chapter and the following exercise, you'll be able to fall into a deep sleep naturally.

And you can get rid of those sleeping pills forever.

The *Naturally Well Relaxation Technique* Script

This method of relaxation has proven itself valuable to people who have trouble unwinding and getting to sleep.

I suggest you record the following script using your own voice in a soothing, lullaby-like manner. You may wish to use peaceful, relaxing music in the background. Play it each night before you go to bed. Gradually, you will learn to relax automatically when the very images contained in the text are brought to mind.

You can also just read rather than record this script, in the same manner, slowly and rhythmically with music in the background. It's not as good as passively listening to a prerecorded session, but it can be effective.

Before you begin, go to the bathroom, empty your bowels and bladder and sit comfortably in a chair or lie on a bed. If you are doing this exercise at night, you should be all ready for bed so you can drift off to sleep as it occurs naturally.

Speak clearly and slowly into your microphone:

I begin by taking three deep breaths. One, all the way in and out; another deep breath . . . two, all the way in and out . . . slower now, and as I take this next breath, all tension is leaving my body.

I am beginning to relax more and more. I relax every part of my body as I ask myself to do so. The deeper I go into a relaxed state of mind and body, the better I feel.

I am beginning to feel a relaxation sensation starting in the toes of both feet, actually feeling it move up to the balls of the feet, to the arches, to the heels, up to the ankles, and I am beginning to feel so relaxed and peaceful, so peaceful.

The relaxation power is now moving up, up to the knees, and I feel calm and very relaxed, my muscles are loose and limp, loose and limp.

The relaxation sensation is now moving up from the knees to the hips and I feel the thigh muscles letting go. Letting go, more and more. And I feel the relaxation moving up into the hip muscles. Relaxing the muscles . . . letting go.

This relaxation sensation permeates every cell, every atom of my body, relaxing me completely, relaxing me completely.

The relaxation power is now moving up to the abdomen, causing the stomach muscles to let go, more and more . . . letting go . . . relaxing the stomach muscles.

It is now moving up to the muscles of my chest, and I feel my body getting more and more relaxed as I ask myself to do so. The muscles around the chest wall are letting go, allowing me to breathe deeply, fully, as I drift into a wonderful feeling of peace and contentment.

This sensation is now moving up into the shoulders, down both arms to the elbows, to the fingers. I feel it as it moves down the arms to the fingers . . . a warming sensation . . . relaxing me completely.

I am now beginning to feel the relaxation sensation moving down my back, gliding so slowly down the muscles of my back. The muscles along both sides of the spine are relaxing, letting go, letting go.

I am beginning to feel this relaxation sensation moving into the neck. The muscles of the neck are letting go, effortlessly.

I feel the scalp muscles letting go, more and more and more. As I am going into a very relaxed state of mind and body, I feel the relaxation power affecting the muscles of the forehead and the facial muscles.

The jaw muscles are relaxing, allowing a little space between the teeth; even the throat is relaxed and softening.

I'm going to count to 25 and on the count of 25, I will be in a very deep, relaxed state of mind and body.

(Speak very slowly) One . . . , two . . . , deeper and deeper; three . . . , four . . . , five . . . , deeper and deeper; six . . . , seven . . . , eight . . . , now deeper and deeper; nine . . . , ten . . . , eleven . . . , relax more and more; twelve . . . , thirteen . . . , fourteen . . . , deeper and deeper; fifteen . . . , sixteen . . . , seventeen . . . , deeper; eighteen . . . , nineteen . . . , twenty . . . , relax more and more; twenty-one . . . , twenty-two . . . , twenty-three . . . , totally relaxed; twenty-four . . . , twenty-five.

I now imagine myself walking through a beautiful meadow, actually experiencing the sounds, the sensual aromas of nature. And as I walk through the meadow I remove my shoes and I feel my feet on the soothing grass and it feels like cotton, so soft and so warm.

It's a beautiful, sunny day, and as I lie down on the grass, I can feel the sun gently warming my entire body. I feel very peaceful and calm. I can hear the sound of water gently bubbling nearby which relaxes me even more. The fragrance of the meadow flowers floats by on the breeze. The wind gently moves the meadow grass back and forth, back and forth, allowing me to be totally peaceful and relaxed.

As I am lying here in the meadow, I can see a patch of clouds moving across the sky, so slowly, and I am feeling so relaxed and peaceful. So peaceful.

I am beginning to feel each part of my body becoming healthier. I am feeling better than I have ever felt before. Much more relaxed; healthier than I have ever felt before.

I see myself lying down in the meadow, content, healthy, happy, peaceful, and as I see myself in that state of mind and body, I'm feeling healthier and happier than I have ever felt before, more and more.

Each time I put myself into this content, relaxed, healthy state of mind, my body remembers the pleasant sensations I am now feeling. Should I wish to recall this relaxed feeling in my day to day activities, I remind myself of this moment, and immediately this wonderful sensation washes over my mind and my body.

In this relaxed state of mind l have much more real energy than I've ever had before.

I'm becoming healthier and happier. Much more productive. Each day, as I hear these words, I feel myself getting healthier and happier, more relaxed, more dynamic, as I am connecting with a deep reservoir of peacefulness and natural strength within me.

All activities are done in a relaxed mindful state and I have no need to use excessive energy to carry out day-to-day tasks.

I have more than enough energy for the body to heal itself. I feel better than I've ever felt before. Totally relaxed, totally relaxed.

As I listen to myself speaking these words at bedtime, I begin to move into a deep, natural, wonderful sleep.

(You may want to say the following sentence rather than the previous one if you are doing this relaxation procedure for a quick pick-me-up during the day).

Should I be listening to these words at the office or elsewhere that needs me to be fully attentive, I count to 5 and I am fully conscious, having much more energy than I ever have had before. One . . . , two . . . , three . . . , four . . . , five . . . .

I am totally happy, healthy and relaxed . . . .

Please remember, never listen to a relaxation audio program while you are driving or doing anything that demands your full attention.

You may also want to visit *www.PsynchroMind.com* to purchase a CD or a downloadable audio program to help you relax and get into a deep sleep, naturally.

7

Psychoimmunity or How to Get Well at the Bates Motel

Modern research has repeatedly shown that resistance to disease not only has roots in the physical body, but also in the emotional and mental states we consistently experience. This is known as psychoimmunity (or psychoneuroimmunology).

In other words, our health is not only determined by what's been discussed in previous chapters about nutrition, rest and exercise, but also by our predominant emotional attitudes about our life and the world around us. Our thoughts and feelings can be 'healers or slayers' depending on the attitudes we choose to adopt.

In the first chapter we discussed how we can manifest into our life that which we worry about most. By focusing on unpleasant things, events and people, we can develop a mindset where we perceive the glass as always 'half empty.' If we keep that view, over time, this negativity will move from the mind to the body, suppressing our ability to enjoy optimal health. Therefore, if our self-scripted biography (our life story and the meaning we give it) is mostly pessimistic, it can become our biology. Our thoughts can literally make us sick.

This chapter may be the most important one in this book because it's about attitude, it's about keeping promises we make to ourselves and it's about realizing that we as individuals must manage, guide and influence our own health and destiny. There's no one else who can do it for us.

If you have problems in your life–with your job, your relationship, an unhealthy habit, a health issue–perhaps you can change your perception of that problem and then it becomes less of a problem. However, I understand how easy that is to say but quite another to implement, especially when you are so close to and immersed in a difficult situation.

What I'm advising is that you look at any unpleasant situation as it exists and try to seek healthy options to deal with it. And if you can't, well, then, there's not much you can do about it. Worrying and fretting about it won't fix the problem, so relax and focus on what you want to have happen. Things usually have a way of working themselves out.

My way of dealing with a problem is to try my best and then let go. If it's meant to be solved it will be solved. If not, there's a reason for the stuck situation that usually reveals itself in time.

Just be aware that a prolonged state of unhappiness actually causes the immune system to malfunction; in extreme cases it might break down altogether. And yes, in turn, will leave you wide open to a myriad of diseases.

It therefore makes sense to work at your personal happiness consistently without adopting a Pollyanna complex. You have to be able to see reality as it is, but not worse than it is. In this frame of mind, you can begin to do something about your problems.

What's really exciting about the field of psychoimmunity is there is so much written about this topic in medical literature with documented case histories of how attitude affects a person's health.

Some people who are terminally ill and told they only have six months to live, have abandoned their former lifestyles and really lived life to the fullest. Some of them found joy in things they would never have considered doing or experiencing before their diagnosis. And the magical side to this is that people have actually lived many years longer than their prognosis. Some have even cured themselves.

Many hospitals now have complementary medical departments that offer massage, healing touch energy therapies and visualization techniques. They teach patients how to enter into relaxation or meditative states and visualize the body healing itself, but in specific and maybe rather unorthodox ways. For instance, one person might visualize that polar bears are inside the body eating up the cancer cells. This image helps change a patient's mindset from that of victim to fighter.

Because the mind and body are so interconnected, doctors are finding that when you focus intensely and repeatedly on something long enough, these kinds of mind-body therapies have measureable results.

The significance of emotional factors cannot be discounted in medicine, and more and more people are discovering that attitudinal imbalances create physical imbalances. Disease is a chain reaction. Why are we sick? Were sick because we don't eat properly. Why don't we eat properly? Because we don't want to look after ourselves. Why don't we look after ourselves? Because we're too busy worrying.

The cause of this is erroneous thinking and it always works against us.

When you improve your attitude, things begin to change. Attitude is like a magnet; you begin to attract people who are happier and you begin to attract situations that are better for you. Lo and behold, your whole world starts to open up. Seems too simplistic, too good to be true, you say? I challenge you to try it for a week and see what happens.

To determine how positive or negative your thoughts are, do 'thought checks' throughout the day; stop what you are doing at 10 a.m. and 2 p.m. and at 5 p.m. and just before you go to bed and see what you were thinking. If you have a cell phone with a built-in alarm, set the alarm and, upon hearing the beep, stop and take stock of what you're thinking at that moment. What are the quality of your thoughts? Are they productive and empowering or just a waste of time and energy?

Most people are very surprised at how much worry, doubt and fear creep into their daily thinking. And if we accept all this doubt, fear and negativity we can get sick, especially if our diet is poor and we don't exercise.

We all have an Aunt Maude. She's the one who constantly complains about being sick and regales family gatherings with her talk of trips to the doctor, the diagnoses, the needles that were stuck in her rear end, the whole gory details. All she talks about is her illness, and if she didn't have that to talk about she'd be speechless. Her illness gives her some importance and it's her way of getting attention.

I often see this happening in relationships. Illness is one way a person can demand attention from a partner. It works. Every time they get sick they get attention. When they aren't sick they don't get the attention. This is one way we can bring illness upon ourselves.

In my experience, some people seem to never seem to want to get well. There is a self-defeating part of them that wants to stay sick for their own reasons. Most of this resistance to becoming well is unconscious, because often they really do want to be healthy and enjoy life fully. At least this is what they say.

I used to see this with insurance claimants who had been involved in car accidents. Those forced to keep a 'pain diary' by insurance companies could prolong their distress because they had to focus on where and when they hurt every day of the week for many months. Note that the more real or imaginary pain they recorded, the bigger the expected payout. Again, if you focus on what isn't working or what doesn't feel right, say it and believe it long enough, it can stay 'broken.'

Once I had a patient who had ulcerative colitis—an inflammation of the bowel where you excrete blood and mucus. I could see this patient had a lot of resistance and I told her so, because every response to a suggestion was a "Yes, but . . . ". However, she finally agreed to listen to me without interrupting because she said she was desperate to get well.

After her consult and exam, I gave her a list of herbs to purchase that would help begin the healing of her illness. When I told her that the location where she could purchase them was about 20 minutes away, she said she didn't have the time to go.

"You've been sick for four years, passing blood and mucus, and you're telling me that a 20 minute drive is too far away?," I said.

I have seen people get well from such diseases. Effectively managing emotional problems (which includes dealing with unconscious saboteurs) and transforming unhealthy habits can help cure illness. But illness returns as soon as people revert to their old lifestyle habits and negative thinking. And they know it themselves. They are the first to admit it.

How do we change our thinking and thus our behavior? *By paying attention to what we consistently think about and the messages we are exposed to. Thoughts control feelings and feelings control behavior.*

When your clock radio turns on in the morning, you wake up to the news of a plane crash, wars being fought, missiles being fired, murders, rapes and suicides. When you pick up your morning paper, you read about these things at breakfast. You haven't been awake half an hour and already you are bombarded with gloomy and pessimistic information. It's no wonder people are so grumpy when they reach the office.

There has been research done linking illnesses with certain personality types. Were all familiar with the person who tries to cram 25 hours into a 24-hour day. These folks can't sit still, can't relax. To them relaxing is a waste of time. They have to be on the go all the time. These are prime candidates for heart disease because to them stress is normal and they often don't make the time to sit down and enjoy a healthy meal, schedule regular exercise or read a book. They have busy, busy thoughts and may not be focused enough on the quality of their life.

Some people think that aging is automatically related to illness. They read about this connection everywhere. Don't believe it. There are plenty of healthy-living older folks who do quite well with little or no medications or surgeries.

Why shouldn't you be healthy into your 50s, 60s, 70s, 80s and 90s? There are people out there who are doing quite well into retirement and beyond; they exercise, they eat healthy, they are creative and active. These folks are dynamic and vital in their 'old age', expressing more enthusiasm than some younger people half their age. To illustrate this point, I like this story: A doctor tells a rather spry elderly man that his knee hurts because of his age and the old fellow reminds the doctor that his other knee is the same age and it's just fine!

We've all seen people who start acting their chronological age as society perceives them—it's another mindset. Men in their 70s start getting out from a chair like old men and they begin to stoop like old men. Straighten up, if there's nothing physically wrong with you. If you move your body more agilely and think like a younger person, you become younger.

It's incredible how some people buy into an image of how they should behave. For example, some new parents become willing prisoners in their own home. Others strap their kids to their backs and head out for an invigorating walk.

We unwittingly limit ourselves by accepting ridiculous ideas as gospel. People are freaked out by thinking outside the box and fear change because it strays from the status quo. Are there changes that you *know* you must make in your life but you don't because of this fear?

Are you rigidly following the status quo because you haven't taken the time to examine and question it? Try and think things through logically. For example, if your doctor tells you to take aspirin to cure your headaches, think about it. Does it make sense to you? Are headaches the result of a lack of aspirin in the body? Is it possible that the cause lies somewhere else?

Once you dump this fixed image or inflexible way of doing something you'll get a wonderful sense of freedom. You'll be more creative, more spontaneous and you'll have more control over your life.

But beware–this attitude can be infectious. And it may better your life in more ways that you ever could have imagined!

Some people whether young or old, have a magnetic spark of life; they have lots of energy and people love to be around them. At a party, you probably notice that everyone gravitates towards those folks who exude enthusiasm, vitality and zest. Try to be like them in your own way.

Follow through on the guidelines set forth in *Naturally Well*. You can do this. It doesn't have to be hard or complicated. Just make a commitment to do the things that make sense to you. Be patient with yourself and take the first step to better health by doing better. Raise your personal standards and expect more from yourself than anyone else expects from you.

Then, one day, you may notice that you have shifted your behavior just a little. You will realize that this moment is your magnificent beginning, your first step towards a brand new life, one that will be more rewarding than you could ever imagine.

Epilogue

All's Well That Ends Well

To reap the benefits of a completely healthy lifestyle, free of addictive and/or toxic substances (drugs, white sugar and synthetic foods for example), you will need to be conscientious about following the guidelines in this book.

The *Naturally Well* regimen cannot be practiced halfheartedly if you expect to see optimal results. And it's something that you just can't do for a couple of days and then give up. You'll begin to feel a lot better within a few weeks by following the guidelines in this book. Stay on the program even longer and the results will increase exponentially. You don't have to follow this program perfectly, but you must do your best. Start with an initial pledge of just 30 days.

This book is more than just another guide to diet and health; it's a book about commitment–commitment to proper nutrition, adequate rest, regular exercise and a positive mental attitude. By following this new healthier way of living, you will have more energy to apply to a renewed or developing sense of purpose. You will achieve an improved capacity for self-direction.

You will begin to look forward to getting up in the morning and enjoying the things you may now take for granted: making breakfast, walking in the park, going on an outing with your children. By turning everything into something special, in return you will create a happier environment for you and those around you.

I can guarantee that most people who follow the principles outlined in this book will improve their health and their general well-being. They'll eliminate causes and symptoms of many illnesses.

In addition to feeling better, this regimen will make you a smarter consumer; you will be more concerned about the food you buy and you'll start reading package labels to see what's really being put into the food you and your family eat. You'll begin to realize what garbage is being thrust at you through advertisers and fast food outlets, and you'll wonder how you ever let anyone take advantage of you this way.

When you begin to feel genuinely healthy you'll no longer find the same difficulty giving up habits like alcohol, cigarettes, drugs and caffeine. And your ability to give up your dependency on such substances will make you stronger not just physically, but mentally as well.

As this new strength and attitude emerges, you will begin receiving positive responses from your friends, family and coworkers. Your newfound optimism will enable you to feel empowered. You can take charge and direct the course of your life towards your highest purpose.

You are not alone when you worry about the downwards spiral our society is taking. People the world over are just as concerned. Many are refusing to allow the corporate food, pharmaceutical and medical industries (and several government agencies) to entice them down the garden path to ill-health and unhappiness. They are deciding that enough is enough.

Once you commit yourself to this wonderful lifestyle, you will be astonished at how many other people are changing theirs too.

You may seem alone at first, but don't despair. Don't give in to peer pressure. Stick to your guns. If you've decided to stay away from red meat, sugar and alcohol for example, don't be suckered in by anyone's pleas or temptations, no matter how well-intentioned they might be. You have a responsibility to your body and it's counting on you to stand your ground.

Strive to better yourself. In this world, how is it possible that people can be bored? There are so many exciting courses available at community colleges and universities, so many incredible events and exhibits happening each day most likely right around the corner from where you live. Find out where they are and get involved. Many of them are free!

Strive to be an interesting person. When you make your life interesting, exciting and adventurous, opportunities will show up to help you grow into the best person you were meant to be.

There is purpose for your existence on this planet.

Observe, question and savor your life to the fullest.

For more information and guidance, please visit:

www.SuperNaturallyWell.com

This site is dedicated to the products and services pertaining to the 'Supernaturally Well' healing philosophies, techniques, and strategies for optimal living.

SuperNaturally Well emphasizes the integration of body, mind and environment to maximize internal vitality and attention management resources.

www. PsynchroMind.com

PsynchroMind is specifically devoted to helping people overcome and transform self-defeating and self-limiting patterns of behavior.

By using a combination of sensory entrainment audio programs and what we call *Authentic Living Principles*, change can happen in the unconscious mind, the real source of decision making and personal empowerment.

www.NextStepNewLife.com

Next Step*New Life is an interactive gathering place for people looking for concrete answers to their health concerns. It's also for those individuals or families who want to take the 'next step' to attain a higher level of wellbeing.

Most importantly, the Next Step * New Life membership community is where you'll find the warm comfort of others who are searching for reliable and practical information, just like you. You'll find natural healing resources and ideas in the blogs, articles, videos and forum that will help provide the information you seek in a safe environment.

Dr. Randall Hardy

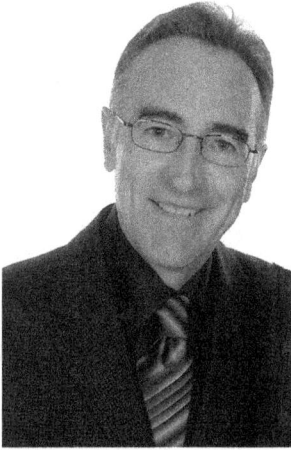

Dr. Randall Hardy is a passionate speaker, health coach and author. His previous careers in chiropractic and naturopathic drugless therapy have given him years of clinical experience to help people enrich their lives and improve their health.

He has also worked and lectured at destination health resorts–educating, motivating and inspiring people to make effective lifestyle changes.

Dr. Hardy has certifications in NLP and medical hypnosis. He has spoken at and sponsored seminars in the US, Canada and the Caribbean.

Randall specializes in safe, natural health care and weight management, disease prevention, stress reduction and the psychology and physiology of motivation and addiction.

Randall is also a member of the National Speakers Association (USA).

Notes:

86

www.ingramcontent.com/pod-product-compliance
Lightning Source LLC
Chambersburg PA
CBHW050555280326
41933CB00011B/1854